A WOMAN'S HEALTH PLANNER

QMP

QUALITY MEDICAL PUBLISHING, INC.

ST. LOUIS, MISSOURI

Cover Art: Back of Nude. *Chase, William Merritt (1849-1916). American. White House, Washington, DC.*

Illustrations courtesy of SuperStock, Inc., Jacksonville, Florida.

Design by Diane Beasley Design.

The information contained in this book is designed to help you make informed decisions about your health. It is not intended as a substitute for medical care. If you suspect that you have a medical problem, you should seek the advice of a medical professional.

Printed in the United States of America.

Quality Medical Publishing, Inc.
11970 Borman Drive, Suite 222
St. Louis, Missouri 63146

ISBN 1-57626-092-5

Contents

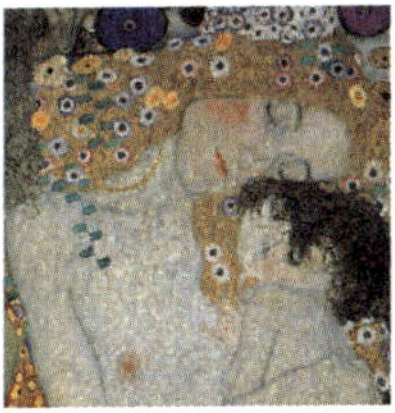

Medical Record

Monitoring Your Health

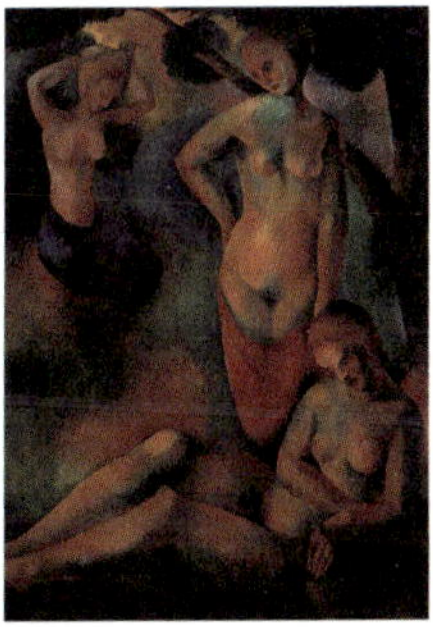

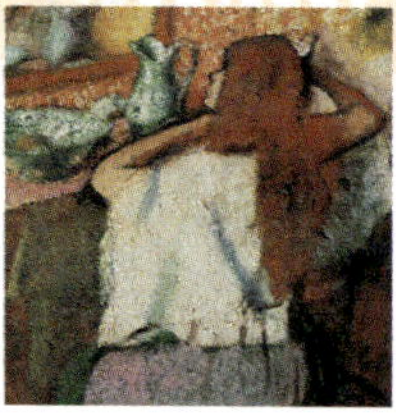

Health Issues

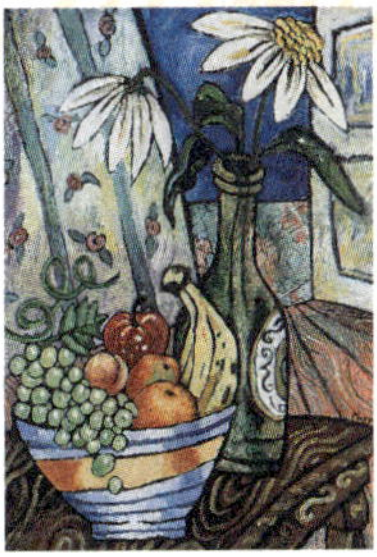

Diet & Nutrition

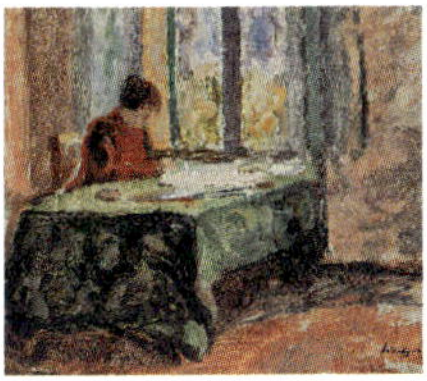

Calendar

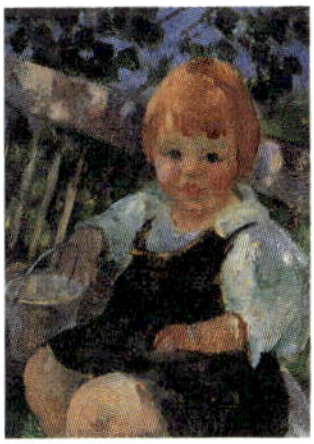

Kids' Notes

Telephone Numbers

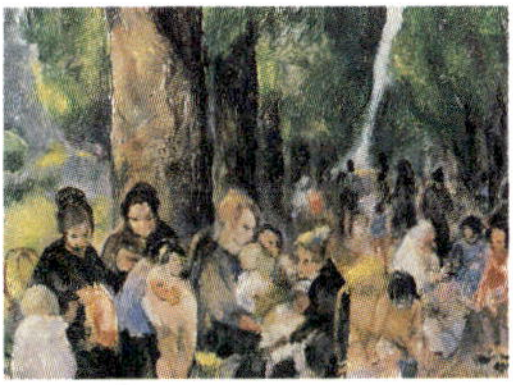

How we spend
our days is,
of course,
how we spend
our lives.

ANNIE DILLARD

Medical Record

Medical Record

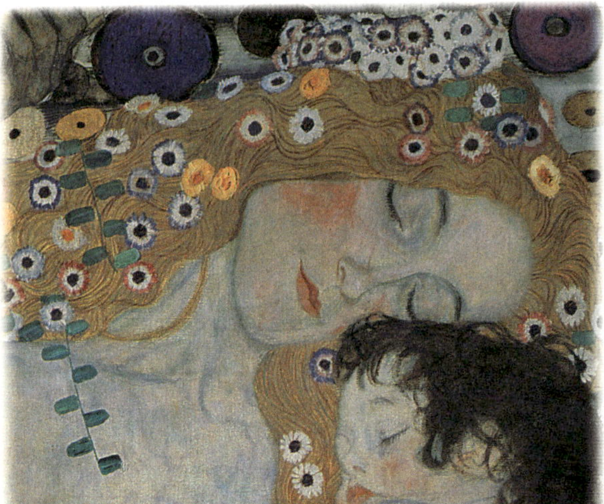

The Three Ages of Woman (detail)

Klimt, Gustave (1862-1918)
Austrian
Gallery of Modern Art
Rome, Italy

Personal Medical Notes

NAME:

BLOOD TYPE:

ALLERGIES:

MEDIC-ALERT:

SOCIAL SECURITY #:

PHYSICIAN:

PHONE:

DENTIST:

PHONE:

EYE DOCTOR:

PHONE:

PHARMACY:

PHONE:

INSURANCE INFORMATION

PLAN:

GROUP #:

NAME OF INSURED:

CLAIMS PHONE #:

In Case Of Emergency Notify

NAME:

STREET:

CITY:

PHONE:

BUSINESS:

ADDRESS:

PHONE:

Family Medical Notes

NAME:

BLOOD TYPE:

ALLERGIES:

MEDIC-ALERT:

SOCIAL SECURITY #:

PHYSICIAN:

PHONE:

DENTIST:

PHONE:

EYE DOCTOR:

PHONE:

PHARMACY:

PHONE:

INSURANCE INFORMATION

PLAN:

GROUP #:

NAME OF INSURED:

CLAIMS PHONE #:

In Case Of Emergency Notify

NAME:

STREET:

CITY:

PHONE:

BUSINESS:

ADDRESS:

PHONE:

Family Medical Notes

NAME:

BLOOD TYPE:

ALLERGIES:

MEDIC-ALERT:

SOCIAL SECURITY #:

PHYSICIAN:

PHONE:

DENTIST:

PHONE:

EYE DOCTOR:

PHONE:

PHARMACY:

PHONE:

INSURANCE INFORMATION

PLAN:

GROUP #:

NAME OF INSURED:

CLAIMS PHONE #:

In Case Of Emergency Notify

NAME:

STREET:

CITY:

PHONE:

BUSINESS:

ADDRESS:

PHONE:

KIDS' MEDICAL NOTES

NAME:

BLOOD TYPE:

ALLERGIES:

MEDIC-ALERT:

SOCIAL SECURITY #:

NAME:

BLOOD TYPE:

ALLERGIES:

MEDIC-ALERT:

SOCIAL SECURITY #:

NAME:

BLOOD TYPE:

ALLERGIES:

MEDIC-ALERT:

SOCIAL SECURITY #:

NAME:

BLOOD TYPE:

ALLERGIES:

MEDIC-ALERT:

SOCIAL SECURITY #:

INSURANCE INFORMATION

PLAN:

GROUP #:

NAME OF INSURED:

CLAIMS PHONE #:

PEDIATRICIAN:

PHONE:

DENTIST:

PHONE:

EYE DOCTOR:

PHONE:

PHARMACY:

PHONE:

In Case Of Emergency Notify

NAME:

STREET:

CITY:

PHONE:

BUSINESS:

ADDRESS:

PHONE:

KIDS' MEDICAL NOTES

NAME:

BLOOD TYPE:

ALLERGIES:

MEDIC-ALERT:

SOCIAL SECURITY #:

NAME:

BLOOD TYPE:

ALLERGIES:

MEDIC-ALERT:

SOCIAL SECURITY #:

NAME:

BLOOD TYPE:

ALLERGIES:

MEDIC-ALERT:

SOCIAL SECURITY #:

NAME:

BLOOD TYPE:

ALLERGIES:

MEDIC-ALERT:

SOCIAL SECURITY #:

INSURANCE INFORMATION

PLAN:

GROUP #:

NAME OF INSURED:

CLAIMS PHONE #:

PEDIATRICIAN:

PHONE:

DENTIST:

PHONE:

EYE DOCTOR:

PHONE:

PHARMACY:

PHONE:

In Case Of Emergency Notify

NAME:

STREET:

CITY:

PHONE:

BUSINESS:

ADDRESS:

PHONE:

NOTES

Monitoring Your Health

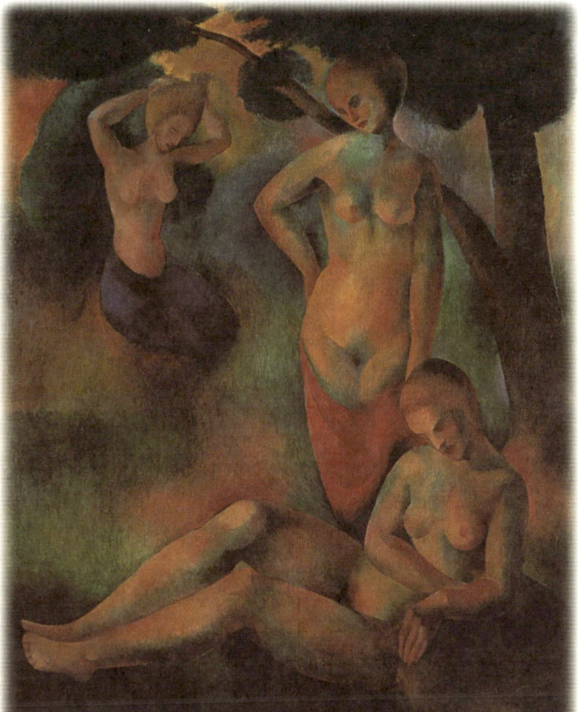

Three Women in a Landscape

Gunschmann, Karl
Christie's
London

Monitoring Your Health

Knowing What To Do in an Emergency

•

Locate area hospitals with 24-hour emergency care.

•

Know (in advance) which hospital or medical facility is nearest your home and office, and tell family and friends to call this facility in an emergency.

•

In addition to this planner keep a list of emergency rescue service numbers next to the telephone and in your wallet or purse.

•

Emergency Numbers

HOSPITAL: ____________________

EMERGENCY RESCUE SQUAD: ____________________

FIRE DEPARTMENT: ____________________

POLICE DEPARTMENT: ____________________

Screening Tests for Women

The following is a compilation of screening recommendations for healthy women without symptoms. Women at high risk for particular disorders may be advised by their physicians to begin certain tests earlier, have them more frequently, or supplement them with other tests.

TYPE OF TEST	COVERED BY INSURANCE?	PREMENOPAUSAL YEARS (35-45)
BLOOD PRESSURE	Yes, if office visit is covered	With every exam (or once a year)
PELVIC EXAM	Yes	Every year
PELVIC-FLOOR MUSCLE STRENGTH	Yes	Every 3-5 years
PAP SMEAR	Check with insurance carrier	Every year
FSH BLOOD TEST	Yes	If you have menopausal symptoms
BREAST EXAM BY PHYSICIAN (SELF-EXAMS MONTHLY)	Yes	Every year
MAMMOGRAM	Yes, in most states; check with insurance carrier	Baseline test before 40; then every 3 years
LIPID PROFILE (CHOLESTEROL SCREEN)	Check with insurance carrier	Baseline test at 35; then every 5 years
DIGITAL RECTAL EXAM	Yes	Every year
STOOL TEST (OCCULT BLOOD)	Check with insurance carrier	Every year after age 40
DENTAL EXAM	Check with insurance carrier	Every 6-12 months (x-rays every 2-3 years)
EYE EXAM (VISUAL ACUITY AND GLAUCOMA)	Check with insurance carrier	
ELECTROCARDIOGRAM	Check with insurance carrier	Baseline at age 40

PERIMENOPAUSAL YEARS (45-55)	POSTMENOPAUSAL YEARS (55-65)	LATER YEARS (65 AND OLDER)
With every exam (or once a year)	With every exam (or once a year)	With every exam (or once a year)
Every year	Every year	Every year
Every 3-5 years	Every year	Every year
Every year	Every year	Every year
If you have menopausal symptoms	If you take postmenopausal hormones, to determine biological efficacy	
Every year	Every year	Every year
Yearly or every 2 years until 50; then every year	Every year	Every year
Every 3 years until menopause	Every other year	Every other year
Every year	Every year	Every year
Every year	Every year	Every year
Every 6-12 months (x-rays every 2-3 years)	Every 6-12 months (x-rays every 2-3 years)	Every 6-12 months (x-rays every 2-3 years)
Every 3 years	Every 3 years	Every 2 years
Per doctor's recommendation	Repeat at age 60	Per doctor's recommendation

Warning Signs You Can't Ignore

If you experience any of these signs, call 911 or your local emergency rescue squad right away. If you can get to a hospital faster by not waiting for an ambulance, the American Heart Association advises that someone drive you there.

HEART ATTACK

- Uncomfortable pressure, fullness, squeezing, or pain in the center of the chest lasting more than a few minutes or occurring intermittently
- Pain spreading to the shoulders, neck, or arms
- Chest discomfort with lightheadedness, fainting, sweating, nausea, or shortness of breath

Not all of these warning signs occur with every heart attack. If some appear, however, don't wait.

STROKE

- Sudden weakness or numbness of the face, arm, or leg on one side of the body
- Sudden dimness or loss of vision, particularly in only one eye
- Loss of speech or problems with talking or understanding speech
- Sudden severe, unexplained headaches
- Unexplained dizziness, unsteadiness or sudden falls, especially along with any previous symptoms

MIGRAINES AND STROKE

In addition to making you miserable, migraine headaches may also indicate a higher risk for stroke. It is not yet known whether reducing the frequency of migraines helps protect against stroke. Still, anyone who suffers from migraines naturally wants to minimize them. Here are some potential triggers:

- Stress.
- Low blood sugar that often accompanies hunger. If your blood sugar is low, a high-protein, low-carbohydrate diet with many small meals during the day may reduce the frequency of migraines.
- Some foods to avoid are aged cheeses, chocolate, hot dogs, deli products, bacon, beer, yogurt, sauerkraut, and yeast. Red wine, MSG, and sudden withdrawal from coffee are also culprits.

BE A HEART SAVER

- If you're with someone experiencing the signs of a heart attack—and the warning signs last more than a few minutes—act immediately.
- Expect "denial." It's normal for someone with chest discomfort to deny the possibility of something as serious as a heart attack. But don't take "no" for an answer. Insist on taking prompt action.
- Call the emergency service or get to the nearest hospital emergency room that offers 24-hour emergency cardiac care.
- Give CPR (mouth-to-mouth breathing and chest compression) if it's necessary and you're properly trained.

Source: American Heart Association, *1994 Heart and Stroke Facts.*

General Symptoms Caused by Different Types of Cancer

- Persistent tiredness for no obvious reason
- Progressive loss of weight for no obvious reason
- Progressive paleness of the tongue or fingernail beds, especially if accompanied by fatigue (paleness and fatigue can mean that one is slowly losing blood and hence becoming anemic)
- Persistent loss of appetite
- Fracture of a bone without any obvious trauma (this can be caused by spread of a cancer from any place in the body to a bone)

CANCER OF THE BREAST

- Mass or thickening in breast or armpit
- Marked asymmetry of breast, a change from normal
- Prominent unilateral veins demonstrating a change
- Unexplained discolorations (redness or bruising)
- Peau d'orange (shiny skin, large pores)
- Ulcerations
- Dimpling, puckering, or retraction of skin or areola
- Fixed inversion of nipple that is a change from normal
- Scaling, crusting, or erosion of the nipple or areola
- Changes in surface characteristics (moles or scars after mastectomy)
- Change in nipple direction
- Nipple discharge

CANCER OF THE LUNG

- A persistent cough not associated with a cold or the flu
- Persistent chest pain, which may or may not be related to coughing
- Persistent hoarseness
- Coughing up blood
- Shortness of breath for no apparent reason
- Frequent and persistent respiratory infections, such as bronchitis or even pneumonia

CANCER OF THE STOMACH

- Any persistent and unexplained abdominal pain or discomfort, including indigestion or heartburn
- Vomiting, especially vomiting blood

CANCER OF THE PANCREAS

Cancer of the pancreas is particularly problematic because it frequently does not produce early symptoms. For this reason it is often referred to as "silent" cancer. One should pay particular attention to:

- Persistent pain in the abdomen, particularly if it spreads to the back
- A yellow discoloration of the skin and the whites of the eyes called jaundice (this can be caused by cancer of the pancreas blocking the duct, or tube, through which bile normally flows)
- Persistent loss of appetite
- Persistent nausea

CANCER OF THE COLON AND RECTUM

- Persistent diarrhea or constipation
- Blood in the stool (the blood can be either bright red in color, dark brown, or even black if the blood has aged)
- Stools that are much narrower than normal
- Loss of weight for no apparent reason
- A feeling that bowel is not completely empty
- General discomfort in the stomach area, such as bloating, fullness, cramps, or gas pains

CANCER OF THE BLADDER

- Bleeding with urination, with or without pain

CANCER OF THE LYMPH GLANDS (LYMPHOMA)

- Painless swelling of the lymph glands in the neck, armpits, or groin
- Heavy sweating during the night
- Persistent itching of the skin for no apparent reason
- Red patches developing on the skin
- Persistent and unexplained nausea and vomiting

CANCER OF THE CERVIX OR UTERUS

- Bleeding between normal menstrual periods
- Bleeding after intercourse or after pelvic examination
- A persistent discharge from the vagina

LEUKEMIA IN ADULTS

- Enlarged lymph glands (as described for lymphoma)
- Persistent bone pain
- A tendency to bleed or bruise easily
- A sense of heaviness or fullness under the left ribs from enlargement of the spleen
- Frequent infections anywhere in the body

Warning Signals That Should Be Reported to Your Physician

If you notice any of these warning signals, see your doctor immediately. Only your physician can determine if they are important:

- Unusual bleeding or spotting between menstrual periods
- Change in bowel or bladder habits
- A sore that does not heal
- Thickening or lump in the breast or elsewhere
- Unusual discharge from the nipples
- Indigestion or difficulty in swallowing
- Obvious change in a wart or mole
- Chronic cough or hoarseness

Risk Factors for Developing Breast Cancer

HIGH RISK

- **Age.** About 80% of breast cancers occur in women over 50.
- **Family history.** Women whose mothers, sisters, or daughters have developed breast cancer are more vulnerable.
- **Previous breast cancer.** If breast cancer develops in one breast, the other breast is at increased risk.

RELATIVE RISK

- History of breast cancer in maternal or paternal grandmother, father's sister, or mother's sister
- Excessive exposure to radiation, particularly before age 20
- Early menarche (menstruation begins before the age of 12)
- Birth of first baby after age 30
- Never having borne children (nulliparity)
- Late menopause (after age 55)
- Obesity
- History of some types of fibrocystic change
- Biopsies showing certain benign changes in the breast tissues or mammograms showing small deposits of calcium in the breast
- Estrogen supplements or replacement

Three Ways to Aid in Early Detection of Breast Cancer

SCREENING MAMMOGRAMS (AMERICAN CANCER SOCIETY GUIDELINES)

- First baseline mammogram should be done by age 40.
- After age 40, mammograms should be done every 1 or 2 years until age 50.
- After age 50, mammograms should be done annually.
- Other factors, such as strong family history or previous breast disease, may indicate the need for mammography at an earlier age.

BREAST EXAMINATION BY YOUR PHYSICIAN

Physician examination should be done annually, more frequently for women who have a high-risk status.

BREAST SELF-EXAMINATION (BSE)

Monthly self-examination should be done to familiarize a woman with what is normal for her breasts and to detect changes when they occur. For premenopausal women—do BSE 5 to 7 days after menstruation ends. After menopause—perform BSE on the same day each month.

How To Do Breast Self-Examination

BSE consists of visual inspection and palpation (feeling).

Visual Exam

- Stand in front of a mirror in a well-lighted room with arms relaxed at sides and carefully observe all sides of your breasts for any changes in breast size or shape, swelling, dimpling, or puckering of the skin, nipple changes, skin rash, scaling, or redness. If you notice any of these, report them to your doctor immediately.
- Clasp hands behind head, press hands forward, and check for any changes in shape or contour of breasts.
- Continue checking as you press hands firmly on hips, hunch shoulders, and lean forward slightly.

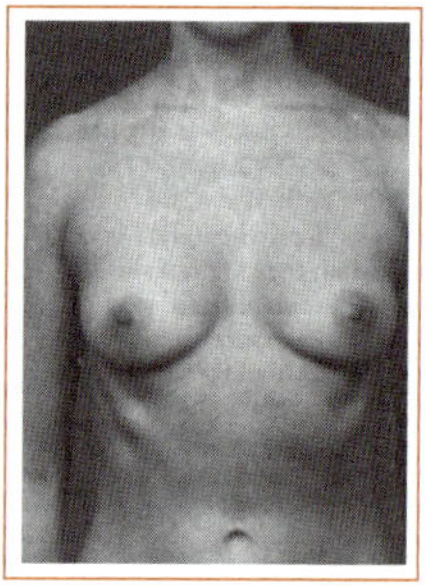

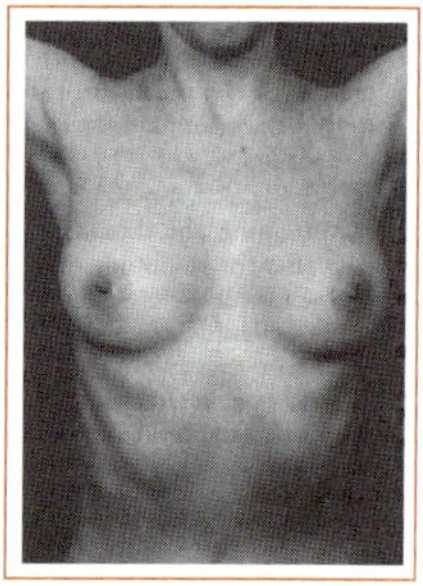

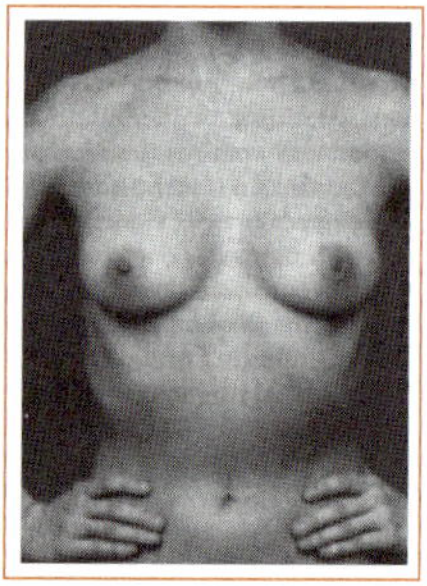

Palpation (Feeling) Exam

- If palpation is performed while standing, begin the inspection by raising your left arm and using the flat, cushioned part of your fingers of your right hand (not the fingertips) to feel your left breast. Place your fingers at the outer edge of your breast, and slowly press or compress the breast tissue gently down to the chest wall beneath. Use one of the three BSE patterns described here. Repeat this exam on your right side. You may want to conduct BSE in the shower, so your fingers can glide over soapy skin and more easily sense changes underneath.
- If you perform the inspection while lying down, lie flat on your back with your left arm over your head and a pillow or rolled towel under your left shoulder. This position flattens your breasts and makes it easier for you to examine them. Use the same palpation, circular, or wedge pattern and repeat the procedure on your right breast.

Patterns for BSE

There are several patterns that you can use for BSE. Select one and use it consistently each month. With all of these patterns, inspect the entire breast region, the areas above the breast and under the collarbone and the underarm, including the armpit itself.

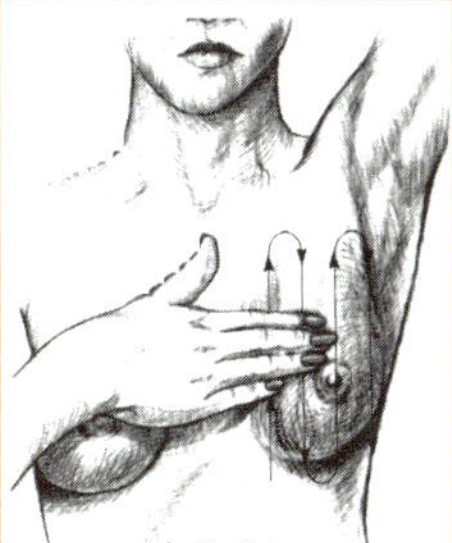

Palpation Pattern

1

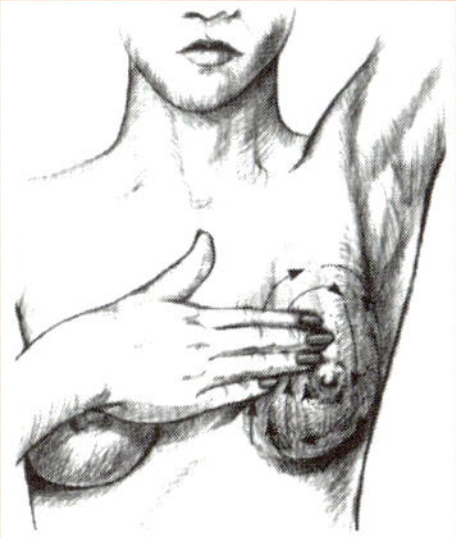

Circular Pattern

2

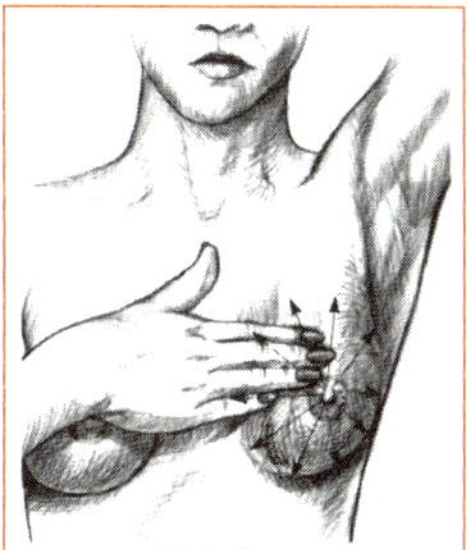

Wedge Pattern

3

1 Move fingers through vertical segments of tissue until the entire breast has been inspected.

2 Begin at outer edge of breast and work in ever-smaller concentric circles, ending at the nipple.

3 Examine by wedges, starting at the outer portion of the breast and working toward the nipple.

Skin Cancer Self-Examination

To check your body for suspicious-looking moles, the Skin Cancer Foundation recommends that you perform the following skin exam every 3 months:

- Examine your face, especially the nose, lips, mouth, and ears, front and back.
- Inspect your scalp, using a blow dryer and mirror to expose each section to view.
- Stand in front of a full-length mirror, begin at your elbows, and scan all sides of your upper arms.
- Next, focus on your neck, chest, and torso, lifting your breasts to view the undersides.
- With your back to the full-length mirror, use a hand mirror to inspect the back of your neck, shoulders, and upper back.
- Still using both mirrors, scan your lower back, buttocks, and backs of both legs.
- Sit down. Prop each leg in turn on a chair or stool. Use the hand mirror to examine your genitals. Check front and sides of both legs, from thighs to toes.

NOTE: You may want to have a dermatologist help you do the first examination so that you can be reassured that freckles and existing moles are normal.

Differentiating a Mole From a Melanoma

According to the American Cancer Society, a normal mole is an evenly colored brown, tan, or black spot in the skin. It may be either flat or raised or round or oval with sharply defined borders. Moles are generally less than 6 mm in diameter (about the size of a pencil eraser) and usually don't change in size, shape, or color for many years. The ABCD rule from the American Cancer Society will alert you to what to look for in a melanoma.

ABCD SIGNS OF MELANOMA

A **Asymmetry.** If you draw a line through a melanoma, the halves do not match.

B **Border irregularity.** The edges are ragged, notched, or blurred.

C **Color.** Pigmentation is not uniform. Shades of tan, brown, and black are present. Red, white, and blue may add to the mottled appearance.

D **Diameter.** Most melanomas are greater than 6 mm in diameter (about the size of a pencil eraser).

OTHER POTENTIALLY HARMFUL SKIN CHANGES

Some skin changes may be early signs of skin cancer and warrant a close watch.

- A persistent scaly red patch with irregular borders that sometimes crusts or bleeds
- An open sore that bleeds, oozes, or crusts and remains open for 3 or more weeks
- An elevated growth with a central depression that occasionally bleeds
- A shiny bump or nodule that is pearly, translucent, pink, red, white, tan, brown, or black
- A white, yellow, or waxy scar-like area that often has poorly defined borders
- A wart-like growth that crusts and occasionally bleeds

Resources

NATIONAL BLACK WOMEN'S HEALTH PROJECT
1237 Ralph Davis Abernathy
Boulevard, NW
Atlanta, GA 30310
(404) 758-9590

NATIONAL CANCER INSTITUTE
Cancer Information Clearinghouse
Office of Cancer Communications
Memorial Sloan-Kettering Cancer
Center
1275 York Avenue
P.O. Box 166
New York, NY 10021
(800) 4-CANCER

NATIONAL DRUG ABUSE AND TREATMENT HOTLINE
(800) 662-4357
(800) 662-9832 (Spanish)

NATIONAL KIDNEY FOUNDATION
30 East 33rd Street
New York, NY 10016
(800) 622-9010

NATIONAL OSTEOPOROSIS FOUNDATION
1150 17th Street, NW
Suite 500
Washington, DC 20036
(202) 223-2226
(800) 223-9994

NATIONAL WOMEN'S HEALTH CENTER (NWHC)
2440 M Street, NW
Suite 201
Washington, DC 20037
(202) 293-6045

NATIONAL WOMEN'S HEALTH NETWORK
1325 G Street, NW
Washington, DC 20005
(202) 347-1140

OFFICE OF DISEASE PREVENTION AND HEALTH PROMOTION
National Health Information Center
P.O. Box 1133
Washington, DC 20013-1133
(800) 336-4797

PMS AND MENOPAUSE SELF-HELP CENTER
101 First Street, Suite 441
Los Altos, CA 94022
(415) 964-7268

WOMEN'S AIDS NETWORK
(415) 864-4376
(800) 367-2437

Y-ME NATIONAL ORGANIZATION FOR BREAST CANCER INFORMATION AND SUPPORT
18220 Harwood Avenue
Harwood, IL 60430
(800) 221-2141
(708) 799-8228 (Illinois)

Health Issues

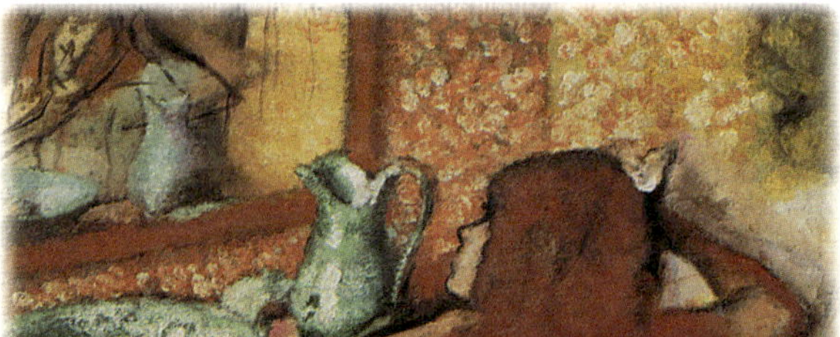

Femme A Sa Toilette

Degas, Edgar (1834-1917)
French
Christie's
London

Health Issues

Solitude is not a luxury. It is a right and a necessity.

No one else will guard my quiet time for me. I have to protect it myself.

Sometimes it helps to know that I just can't do it all.

Perfectionism is self-abuse of the highest order.

Sometimes we just think too much!

My illusion of control is just that . . . an illusion.

Knowing when to quit may be my greatest victory.

My interests enrich my life, but not when I go after them compulsively.

Friends add joy to life. I have to be one to have one.

It is sometimes frightening to trust my intuition. It is always disastrous not to trust it.

What I am looking for is not "out there." It is me.

Signs of Stress

- Nervous habits: biting your nails, pacing, and clenching or grinding your teeth
- Physical symptoms: headaches, backaches, fatigue, digestive problems, sexual or menstrual problems, and increased muscular tension
- Sleep problems: can't get out of bed in the morning
- Lack of concentration and difficulty in making decisions: can't find your keys or remember what you were doing or switch tasks every minute or so without following anything through
- Skipping regular exercise routine
- Guilt feelings about relaxation
- Misusing food, alcohol, or drugs: eating a pint of ice cream to cheer yourself up, having a drink to relax, or taking pills to help you sleep
- Loss of self-esteem, a feeling of worthlessness, or problems with moodiness or depression
- Trouble meeting important deadlines
- Sense of paranoia and an increased sensitivity to criticism
- Harder time being creative or productive
- Tendency to criticize others and be argumentative

Relaxation Techniques

By consciously resting the body and clearing the mind of disturbing thoughts, relaxation techniques stop the brain from sending out messages of danger. The mind sends positive, rather than stressful, messages to the muscles. The real benefit of relaxation is to learn to turn off negative thoughts and give the body a break from the constant onslaught of stress.

EXERCISE #1

- Stand with arms at sides, feet comfortably apart, and breathe out completely. Fix your gaze on a spot on the wall or floor to help keep your balance.
- Breathe in as you bring your arms up in a wide circle to the side and overhead, and raise up on your toes.
- Hold breath for a second as you clasp hands and stretch a little farther up.
- Breathe out while returning arms and lowering heels to floor.
- Repeat three times.

EXERCISE #2

- Sit quietly in a comfortable position.
- Close your eyes.
- Deeply relax all your muscles.
- Breathe in and out through your nose; repeat the word *one* silently to clear your mind of extraneous thought.
- Continue for 10 to 20 minutes.
- When finished, sit quietly with eyes closed for a few minutes, then gradually open them.

The Shortcut to Smoother Fresher Skin

Alpha hydroxy acids (AHAs) are the decade's hottest skin care ingredients. They actually make skin smoother, more radiant, and more even toned. Here is some information and tips on AHAs.

WHAT AHAs DO

AHAs (also called fruit acids) are exfoliators that speed the skin's natural cell-shedding process. Skin becomes finer in texture and better able to retain moisture. Because they "unglue" dead surface cells, AHAs keep pores clearer and reduce breakouts in oily skin. They also attract and hold moisture—so they're good for dry skin, too.

AHA CONCENTRATIONS

To get these benefits, you need a product with an AHA concentration of at least 2% (some products go as high as 8% to 10%). Most labels, however, don't specify the AHA concentration.

WHAT TO LOOK FOR ON THE LABEL

Choose a lotion or cream designed for use after cleansing and before moisturizing. Look for words like *AHA, hydroxy, fruit acids, renewing, revealing, and exfoliating*. Some AHA products contain salicylic acid, an exfoliator that is *not* an AHA but does complement these fruit acids. Bottom line: Forget which acid is which. Don't worry about the concentration. The best way to evaluate an AHA is to try it.

EVALUATING THE EFFECTIVENESS

Your skin should be visibly smoother within 2 weeks. Over the next 2 to 8 weeks you should see more clarity, radiance, and evenness of texture. Fine lines should also appear diminished, although deeper lines and wrinkles will not be affected.

SIDE EFFECTS AND APPLICATION TIPS

AHAs should not sting, but they may cause tingling because they are acids. If you experience pain or significant redness, the product is too strong or you are sensitive to that particular formula. Tingling can be minimized by waiting 15 minutes after cleansing before applying AHA. Skin is more permeable just after you cleanse, so more product may penetrate, delivering more of a bite. You might also try a gentle, non-AHA exfoliating formula or a cosmetic line that lets you start with a lower AHA concentration and work up to a higher one—AHAs seem to make skin less sensitive over time.

SAFETY OF AHAs

Unlike Retin-A, AHAs will not make your skin thinner or more sun sensitive; in fact, they seem to make it appear healthier. Don't worry about acid overkill if you use a line that contains several AHA products. AHA levels in cleansers and toners are usually too low to exfoliate. Let your skin tell you how many products are too many. Don't use AHAs with scrubs or other exfoliators.

COSTS OF AHAs

AHAs do not have to be expensive. Many well-known drugstore brands are among the most reasonably priced and have been confirmed by some of the best research. Avoid brands you've never heard of (with AHAs, it's best to stick with familiar companies that do extensive consumer testing).

GAUGING SUN INTENSITY

The ultraviolet (UV) index that is broadcast nationwide and personal UV monitors (like the new SunWatch II or Sun Cast) make it easy to judge sun intensity and how much protection you need before going outdoors. But there are other easy gauges that can clue you in to the sun's intensity.

- **Shadow length.** When your shadow is longer than you are tall, the sun is lower in the sky and thus less intense. When your shadow is shorter than you are tall, the sun is overhead and most intense, with the highest sunburn potential.
- **Shadow sharpness.** When the sun is intense, your shadow or the shade cast by other objects is deep and dark with sharply defined edges. When the sun is less intense or there is cloud cover, shadows are less deeply colored and their edges are blurry.
- **Cloud cover.** The sun may not look as bright, but up to 60% of UV rays can penetrate through overcast skies. Smog, on the other hand, partially filters solar radiation.
- **Sky color.** Azure, cloudless skies indicate more intense radiation. The deeper blue, the more intense the radiation.
- **Breeziness.** When the wind is calm, so is the water. A still surface reflects a substantial amount of UV radiation, depending on the angle of the sun.
- **Geography.** Thin, high-altitude air is less effective at screening out radiation than the denser air at sea level. For every 1000 feet of altitude, the intensity of UV light increases about 4%.
- **Solar flares.** Radio and TV signal interference, frequent aurora borealis displays, and delays in space shuttle flights are all signs of increased solar activity (often mentioned in the news). The UV intensity can increase as much as 15% during times of solar-surface unrest.

Burn Alert Sun Sensitivity

Some drugs (both prescription and over the counter) can increase sun sensitivity, causing you to burn faster with a more extreme reaction ranging from itchiness to rashes to increased pigmentation. Drugs likely to cause sun sensitivity are oral contraceptives, nonsteroidal anti-inflammatory pain relievers (including ibuprofen), diuretics, antihistamines, coal-tar shampoo, the antibiotic tetracycline, and sulfa drugs. Some foods (limes, lemons, grapefruit, celery, fennel, dill, cashews) can even photosensitize the mouth, lips, and body skin.

SUNLAMP WARNING

UV light from sunlamps in tanning parlors is just as dangerous as UV light outdoors. Studies are showing that the interaction of tanning-bed UV rays (mostly UVA) and subsequent solar UVB radiation may increase skin cancer risk.

EXTRA PROTECTION FROM UV EXPOSURE

UV light scatters and bounces, so you also get significant UV exposure even when you're moving around. Extra protection is provided by brimmed hats, protective sunglasses, and high SPF sunscreen on all areas (even ones you can't see, such as your scalp and the nape of your neck). UV light also can penetrate up to 3 feet of water, so a waterproof sunscreen is recommended for protection.

EYE PROTECTION

Eyelid cancers, conjunctival growths, cataracts, corneal burns, and macular degeneration are occurring more frequently. Good UV blocking sunglasses vastly reduce your risk of developing these. Choose lenses that absorb 99% to 100% of UVA and UVB light and most blue light. Clear UV protective film can be applied to eyeglasses. If you wear contacts, try Precision UV, the first flexible-wear UV-blocking contact lenses.

Changes During the Menstrual Cycle

PREMENSTRUAL SYNDROME (PMS)

PMS is the term for a group of emotional, mental, and physical symptoms that affect many women during the days leading up to a menstrual period. The exact cause is unknown but is thought to be related to hormonal changes. Symptoms include:

- Fluid retention
- Mood changes
- Urinary tract infections
- Weight gain
- Carbohydrate cravings
- Disrupted sleep patterns
- Low tolerance to alcohol
- Increase in heart rate and blood pressure
- Stronger asthma symptoms
- Increased susceptibility to viruses
- Frequent migraines, herpes virus infections, and skin eczema
- Breast tenderness
- Breathlessness
- Visual disturbances
- Numbness in fingers
- Headaches
- Back pain
- Nasal congestion

DURING MENSTRUATION

- Increase in urinary output
- Increase in saliva flow
- Greater alcohol tolerance
- Increase in allergies

THE WEEK AFTER MENSTRUATION

- All five senses intensified
- More restorative sleep
- Body temperature drops below normal (98.6° F) by one half to one degree

DURING OR NEAR OVULATION

- Cervical mucus changes
- Runny and copious vaginal discharge

AFTER OVULATION

- Body temperature rises back up to 98.6° F
- Craving for sweets
- Food intake and energy expenditure rise

Menstrual Problems

DYSMENORRHEA (PAINFUL PERIODS)

Fifty percent of menstruating women suffer low abdominal pain, cramps, backache, and pains in the thighs, sometimes accompanied by nausea, vomiting, and diarrhea. Some form of pain is experienced by 80% of girls under the age of 19. The pains often occur just before menses and can last for 2 days.

AMENORRHEA

When menses (periods) fail to start, or are interrupted, the condition is known as amenorrhea. The most common causes are pregnancy and breast-feeding. Amenorrhea can also be a side effect of being severely underweight or of excessive exercising. It may also result from stress, certain chronic diseases, or the long-term use of some medications.

ABNORMAL PERIODS

Irregular, prolonged, and heavy menses (periods) are most common in adolescence and the years prior to menopause. These are often due to a hormonal imbalance. Menstruation is also influenced by diet, body weight, and activity levels. Irregular menses tend to be related to the level of estrogen in the body. When estrogen levels are low, blood spotting is light but sustained; when levels are high, no bleeding may be followed by profuse blood loss. Prolonged and heavy menses are often the result of low progesterone levels.

TOXIC SHOCK

This is a rare condition, usually linked to the use of tampons left in place for extended periods encouraging excessive growth of normally occurring bacteria *(Staphylococcus aureus)*; the same is true of cervical caps and diaphragms. The bacteria could also have been introduced into the vagina on the fingers. The bacteria produce a toxin that can cause shock, kidney failure, coma, and death. Tampons should always be removed after 4 to 6 hours.

Yeast Infections

Yeast infections affect 80% of all women at some point. They are caused by the yeast *Candida albicans,* which occurs naturally in the bowel. Problems occur when the yeast is able to grow uncontrolled by other organisms, such as often happens following a course of antibiotics.

SYMPTOMS

- Dryness
- Severe itching
- Thick, curdy discharge from the vagina
- Soreness
- A yeasty odor

TREATMENT OPTIONS

If you have had a previously diagnosed yeast infection and are familiar with the symptoms, over-the-counter creams/suppositories are available. Otherwise see your physician for an accurate diagnosis.

Bladder Infections (Cystitis)

Cystitis is an infection in the bladder. It is also known as the "honeymoon disease" (frequent sexual intercourse may prompt an infection), leading to an increased desire to pass urine, as well as severe pain upon urination.

Cystitis requires immediate treatment, not only because it is very painful, but also because the infection can spread to the kidneys. Consult your doctor.

Reduce risk by always wiping or washing from front to back.

URINARY INCONTINENCE

Urinary incontinence refers to the inability to control urine flow, from occasional leakage of a few drops to sudden bursts of flow (stress incontinence) or constant dripping from the urethra. The most common type among women is stress incontinence, in which small amounts of urine leak when you sneeze, cough, or laugh. If you have these symptoms, check with your primary care provider.

KEGEL EXERCISES TO HELP PREVENT URINARY STRESS INCONTINENCE

Kegel exercises strengthen the muscles involved in urination and may help you regain better bladder control. Learn to isolate the muscles involved by starting and stopping your urinary stream. Then practice slowly tightening and releasing these muscles several times a day while sitting or standing. As you become skilled, you should be able to do 20 to 30 repetitions three or four times a day.

TIPS FOR PERFORMING KEGEL EXERCISES

- You can locate your pubococcygeus (PC) muscle by partially emptying your bladder and then squeezing and releasing several times midstream. Be sure to empty your bladder completely after you are done with the exercise to avoid urine retention.
- Once you have located the PC muscle, begin tensing and relaxing it. To check if you are doing this correctly, insert a finger into your vagina and tighten the muscles to squeeze the finger.
- Start doing the Kegel exercises by tensing and then immediately relaxing. Gradually increase the number of repetitions, and then progress to keeping the muscles tense for up to 10 seconds. Some experts recommend doing 100 Kegels a day.
- You can perform Kegels anywhere—while cooking, watching TV, sitting at your desk, waiting for a light to change, standing in an elevator.

Important Facts About Menopause

Menopause occurs gradually. For most women, the changes signaling the approach of menopause begin in the late thirties when the ovaries start producing less estrogen. In the mid-forties, most women experience a decrease in the frequency of ovulation. Between the ages of 45 and 55, periods become irregular in frequency and flow, ushering in the *climacteric* when they come to an end. Menopause has arrived when you haven't had a period for at least a year. Although rare, menopause can occur as early as age 35 or as late as age 60.

SYMPTOMS OF MENOPAUSE

Reduced levels of estrogen can result in many different symptoms. Women vary in the amount and severity of symptoms they suffer, and some symptoms are much more common than others. Of the following symptoms associated with the perimenopause, only hot flashes are uniquely menopausal:

- Headaches
- Hot flashes
- Insomnia
- Sweating
- Dizziness
- Anxiety
- Depression
- Irritability
- Loss of concentration
- Changes in libido
- Urge incontinence
- Vaginal dryness
- Bone aches and pains
- Heavy menses

Coping With Hot Flashes

Hot flashes are one of the first physical signs of menopause and most women experience these flashes to some degree.

Ways to deal with hot flashes that do not involve drugs:

- Dress in layers of light, natural-fiber clothing that can be removed easily.
- Have a cold drink.
- Carry a pretty fan and don't be shy about using it.
- Place a cool washcloth on your forehead, wrists, or temples.
- Stand by an open window (if it's cool outside).
- Keep rooms at a cool temperature. Get an electric blanket with dual controls if you and your partner argue about temperature.
- Sleep with lightweight blankets.
- Take a lukewarm shower if you can.
- Note when flashes occur (i.e., months when you do not menstruate or when you wear a heavy sweater), so you can be better prepared for them.
- Eat foods rich in vitamin E, such as wheat and rice germs, legumes, corn, almonds, vegetable oils, and egg yolks. Consult with your doctor about taking a supplement; many physicians recommend starting with 25 mg a day and gradually increasing the dose to no higher than 400 or 800 mg.
- Cut back on caffeine, alcohol, spicy food, hot soup and drinks, and large meals.
- Keep the room temperature around 68° F.
- Try sitting quietly when you feel a flash coming on. "Visualization" exercises may help reduce the stress these sensations can create—imagine the flash washing harmlessly over you like a wave.

Many women choose hormone replacement therapy to end hot flashes. Women who cannot take estrogen may get some relief from taking progestin.

Osteoporosis

Osteoporosis is a disease marked by loss of bone tissue. More than 25 million Americans suffer from the disease, and about 1.3 million of them will suffer fractures, mostly of the hip, spine, and wrist. Women are generally thinner, have smaller bones, a longer life span, and are more susceptible to developing this condition.

Although we all lose some bone tissue as we age, osteoporosis is not a normal part of getting older. It is, in fact, a preventable disease.

Preventing Osteoporosis

Strong bones require sufficient calcium, which along with proper exercise—particularly resistance weight training—builds up your bone bank.

CALCIUM

- Take daily minimum requirement.

EXERCISE

- Weight-bearing exercise (walking, running, and aerobic dancing), but not swimming or biking, for 45 minutes every other day reduces the risk of osteoporosis, although it probably will not have a significant effect in women not taking estrogen.
- Exercise both the upper and lower body. Weight training, combined with aerobic exercise, ensures an entire body workout.
- Exercises that strengthen the back and abdominal muscles maintain flexibility and improve balance to prevent falls and possible fractures.

SMOKING

Smoking increases the risk of osteoporosis and hip fractures, counteracting the beneficial effects of estrogen on the bones.

Recommended Calcium Intake

Following are the updated American Dietetic Association recommendations for daily calcium intake. Note: Recommendations are now broken into age groups and apply to both men and women. Pregnant women should check with their physicians to ensure that they are getting adequate amounts.

AGE	RECOMMENDED DAILY INTAKE (mg)
1-3 years	500
4-8 years	800
9-18 years	1300
19-50 years	1000
51 and over	1200

Osteoporosis and Prescription Drugs

Osteoporosis experts urge you to check out any prescription drugs you are taking. The following medications can weaken your bones by reducing your body's ability to absorb calcium from food and increasing the amount of calcium excreted in the urine:

- Diuretics
- Anticoagulants (blood thinners used to prevent clots and strokes)
- Steroids, sometimes prescribed to treat arthritis, asthma, lupus, and Crohn's disease

If it is absolutely necessary for you to take these medications, ask your doctor if an alternative drug is available or whether the dosage can be reduced. If you continue taking these drugs for a long time or at high dosages, your doctor may order a bone-density test, which identifies early bone thinning.

TIPS FOR TAKING CALCIUM SUPPLEMENTS

Food is the best source of calcium, but most of our diets don't include adequate daily quantities (the equivalent of about 4 cups of milk) of the mineral. Nutritionists advise making up the shortfall with a supplement.

- Labels on supplements can be confusing. The calcium content of a tablet is usually expressed as the United States Recommended Dietary Allowance (U.S. RDA). To find the milligrams, add zero to the percent listed. Thus a product containing 30% of the U.S. RDA equals 300 mg of calcium.
- To determine how many calcium tablets you need, read the label. The number depends on how much calcium you get from your food sources.
- Not all calcium supplements dissolve adequately enough to be absorbed by your stomach. To test your supplement, place it in a glass of vinegar at room temperature and stir occasionally for 30 minutes. If the tablet hasn't disintegrated, it won't dissolve in your stomach either.
- Stick to the brand-name supplements.
- Plain calcium carbonate is perfectly adequate.
- Do not take bone meal or dolomite calcium supplements, which may contain lead or other toxic metals.
- Calcium is better absorbed in small amounts. Divide your supplements so that you do not take more than 500 mg at one time.
- Take calcium carbonate supplements with meals or at bedtime.
- Talk to your doctor or pharmacist about potential interactions between calcium and prescription and nonprescription medications you are taking.
- Talk to your doctor before taking supplements if you have a personal or family history of kidney stones.
- Do not take iron supplements at the same time; they can interfere with calcium absorption.
- Include calcium-fortified foods in your diet.

Calcium: Selected Good Food Sources

FOOD	SERVING	CALCIUM (mg)
Beans		
white beans, canned	½ cup	96
pinto, canned	½ cup	44
garbanzo (chickpeas) canned	½ cup	39
red kidney, canned	½ cup	31
Cheese		
ricotta, part-skim	4 oz	337
Parmesan, hard	1 oz	336
Swiss	1 oz	272
Monterey Jack	1 oz	212
mozzarella, part-skim	1 oz	207
cheddar	1 oz	204
Muenster	1 oz	203
American	1 oz	174
cottage, low-fat (2%)	4 oz	77
Corn tortilla	1 medium	44
Figs (dried)	3	80
Fish		
sardines, canned in oil, with bones	3½ oz	382
salmon, canned with bones	3½ oz	226
Ice milk, vanilla, soft-serve	1 cup	276
Milk		
skim	8 oz	302
low-fat (1%)	8 oz	300
low-fat (2%)	8 oz	297
whole	8 oz	291
Orange juice (calcium-fortified)	8 oz	300
Tofu (processed with calcium sulfate)	½ cup	260
Vegetables		
turnip greens, cooked	½ cup	99
kale, cooked	½ cup	90
mustard greens	½ cup	75
okra, cooked	8 pods	54
chard, cooked	½ cup	51
broccoli	½ cup	45
fennel, raw	3½ oz	43
Yogurt		
plain, nonfat	8 oz	452
plain, low-fat	8 oz	415
fruit, low-fat	8 oz	345
frozen	½ cup	105

Resources

Resources

Notes

NOTES

Notes

NOTES

NOTES

Diet & Nutrition

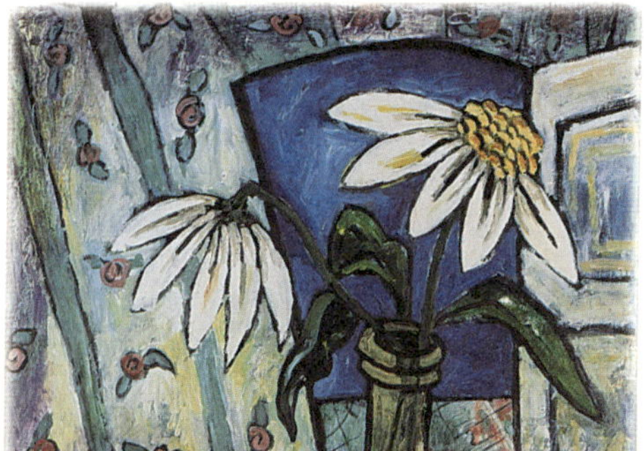

Centerpiece of the Gods

Pierre, Christian
American
Private Collection

WEIGHT LOSS

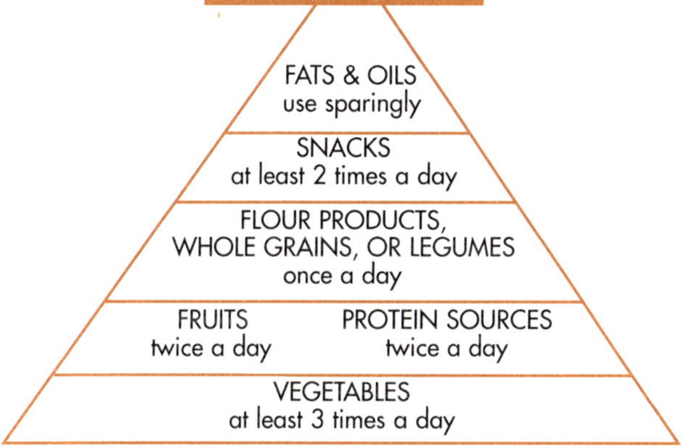

Alcoholic beverages: 2 per week*

MAINTENANCE

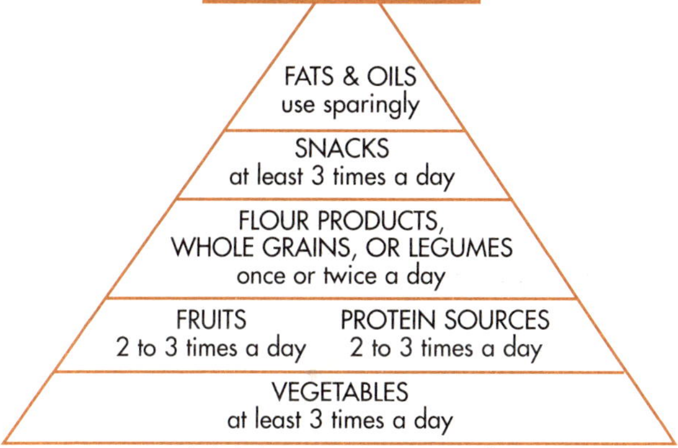

Alcoholic beverages: 3 to 6 per week*

*1 serving = 1 glass of wine or 1 beer or 1 mixed drink

Essential Nutrients

NUTRIENTS	FOOD SOURCES
Protein	Milk, cheese, yogurt, eggs, fish, poultry, meat, beans, tofu
Fats	Whole milk, most cheeses, butter and margarine, oils, nuts, meats
Carbohydrates	Grains and cereals, breads, pasta, fruits, vegetables, beans
Water	Tap and bottled water, coffee, tea, juice, soup, fruits, vegetables
Fiber	Fruits, vegetables, whole-grain breads and cereals, legumes

Essential Vitamins

VITAMIN	FUNCTION	FOOD SOURCES
Vitamin A	Increases resistance to infection; contributes to healthy skin and good vision	Fish liver oil, liver, whole milk, butter, egg yolks, dark green, yellow, and orange fruits and vegetables
Beta carotene	Helps protect against skin and lung cancer	Yellow or orange vegetables
Vitamin B complex	Metabolizes carbohydrates and proteins; helps protect against heart disease; maintains healthy cells, nervous system, skin, and intestines; and is a good source of energy	Whole-grain breads and cereals, liver, wheat germ, green vegetables, lean meats, milk, cheese, peanuts, dried peas and beans, nuts and seeds, eggs, poultry, potatoes, fish, molasses
Folic acid	Synthesizes essential nucleic acids for cell division; promotes formation of red blood cells; helps protect against heart disease; prevents spina bifida	Peas, bananas, nuts, whole-grain breads and cereals
Vitamin C	Essential component of bones, vascular system, muscles, cartilage, tissues; promotes formation of hemoglobin and red blood cells; encourages the body to fight infection and stress	Citrus fruits, sweet peppers, leafy greens, broccoli, cauliflower, tomatoes, fresh potatoes, berries, melons, bean sprouts
Vitamin D	Essential for strong bones and teeth	Sunlight on bare skin, fortified milk, fish liver oil
Vitamin E	Maintains red blood cell tissues; ensures normal muscle metabolism; and is an antioxidant	Vegetable oils, wheat and rice germ, egg yolks, legumes, corn, almonds

Essential Minerals

MINERAL	FUNCTION	FOOD SOURCES
Calcium	Necessary for building strong bones and teeth; blood clotting; regulating nerve and muscle activity; preventing muscle cramps	Milk and milk products, leafy greens, broccoli, artichokes, ground sesame seeds, canned fish containing bones
Iron	Transfers and transports oxygen; important component of hemoglobin	Lean meat, liver, egg yolks, leafy greens, wheat germ, whole-grain and enriched breads and cereals, legumes, oysters, turkey, dried fruit
Magnesium	Helps regulate body temperature, nerve impulses, and muscle contractions; necessary for normal metabolism of calcium and potassium	Whole grains, leafy greens, beans, seafood, nuts
Phosphorus	Helps to metabolize fats and carbohydrates into energy; component of all body cells; necessary for building strong bones and teeth	Milk, cheese, lean meats, eggs, fish, nuts and seeds, poultry, legumes, whole grains, soft drinks
Potassium	Regulates fluid levels in cells; needed for healthy nerves and muscles	Fresh ripe fruits (especially bananas) and vegetables; legumes, fish, poultry, meat, milk
Zinc	Stimulates digestion; aids in extracting stores of vitamin A from the liver; helps maintain the mucous lining of the mouth, throat, stomach, and intestines; vital for the normal growth of hair, skin, and nails; controls sexual maturation and fertility; aids in wound healing	Pumpkin seeds, liver, egg yokes, seafood (especially oysters)

A Prudent Diet for Cancer Prevention

- Maintain a desirable body weight.
- Eat a variety of fruits and vegetables each day.
- Eat plenty of high-fiber foods, such as whole-grain breads and cereals, legumes, fruits, and vegetables.
- Reduce your fat intake to no more than 20% of your daily calories.
- Limit your consumption of alcoholic beverages, if you drink at all.
- Limit your consumption of salt-cured, smoked, and nitrite-preserved foods.

The Anti-Skin Cancer Diet

Wearing sunscreen and avoiding excessive sun exposure are key to preventing skin cancer, but diet may also help save your skin from basal and squamous cell carcinomas, the two most common types of skin cancer. The amount of fat consumed has a direct effect on the development of these tumors. A low-fat diet (no more than 20% of daily calories coming from fats), along with sunscreen use, may dramatically decrease the incidence of skin cancers.

Calculating Your Daily Calorie Needs

Figure your energy requirement by multiplying what you consider your ideal weight by your activity level. If you are:

A	Sedentary	multiply by	13
B	Active	multiply by	15
C	Very active	multiply by	17

(Appropriate body weight) × (Activity level) = Calories/day

If you weigh more than your appropriate weight, add calories; if less, subtract.

(Calories from item B above) − 500 = to *LOSE* 1 pound a week

(Calories from item B above) + 500 = to *GAIN* 1 pound a week

Set your daily goal: _______ calories

Exercise and Calories Burned

How many calories you use when exercising depends on several factors:

- **How much you weigh.** The more you weigh, the more you burn.
- **How long you exercise.** The best way to burn calories is to exercise moderately for a longer time and increase the distance you cover.
- **Air (and water) temperature.** Exercising in cold air or cool water uses extra calories because your body does extra work to keep warm.

Exercise and Calories Burned (cont.)

The following table shows the approximate calories used per minute for various activities by a woman weighing 127 to 137 pounds.

Activity	Calories
Aerobic dancing	6.58
Bicycling	
5.5 mph	3.58
10 mph	6.16
stationary, 10 mph	6.25
Calisthenics	4.50
Gardening, weeding, and digging	5.75
Golf, hand cart	3.75
Hiking, 20-lb pack, 2 mph	4.50
Jogging	
5.5 mph	9.75
8 mph	11.90
Rope jumping	
55 per min	7.58
95 per min	9.75
Rowing machine	
easy	4.50
vigorous	9.75
Sawing wood by hand	5.83
Skiing	
downhill	8.83
cross-country, 5 mph	10.41
cross-country, 9 mph	14.83
Snow shoveling	
light	9.08
heavy	15.66
Stair climbing	
normal	6.70
rapid	14.80
Walking	
2 mph	2.80
4 mph	5.20

Calculating Your Heart Rate

TO DETERMINE YOUR HEART RATE

1 Find your pulse with your fingers.

2 Count the number of beats in 10 seconds.

3 Multiply this number by 6 to determine your heart rate in beats per minute.

HOW TO CALCULATE YOUR TARGET HEART RATE

1 Calculate your approximate maximum heart rate:

220 – Age = Maximum heart rate

2 Multiply this number by 0.6. This number is your lower heart rate limit for aerobic exercise.

3 Multiply your maximum heart rate by 0.8. This number is your upper limit heart rate for aerobic exercise.

4 Your target heart rate range during aerobic exercise is defined by your lower and upper heart rate limits.

TO DETERMINE YOUR RESTING HEART RATE

1 Maximum heart rate (*see above*) minus 85.

A WOMAN AGE 40 WOULD CALCULATE HER HEART RATE AS FOLLOWS:

1 Calculate the maximum heart rate:

$$220 - 40 = 180$$

2 Multiply by 0.6:

$$180 \times 0.6 = 108$$

3 Multiply the maximum rate by 0.8:

$$180 \times 0.8 = 144$$

4 Lower heart rate limit: 108
Upper heart rate limit: 144

Keeping Tabs on Dietary Fat and Cholesterol

A heart-healthy diet is one that is low in saturated fats and cholesterol. Cholesterol is a soft, fat-like substance that travels through the blood stream and is present in all the cells of your body. **Some** cholesterol is essential, but too much increases your risk of heart attack. Saturated fats are the main dietary culprit in raising blood cholesterol. They are found mostly in foods from animals and some plants:

- Beef, beef fat, veal, lamb, pork, lard, poultry fat, butter, cream, milk, cheeses, and other dairy products made from whole milk (because these foods are from animals they also contain dietary cholesterol)
- Coconut oil, palm oil, and palm kernel oil ("tropical" oils), and cocoa butter (because these are extracted from plants they are cholesterol free)

Fats may be hydrogenated during processing to improve texture and lengthen shelf life. Recent studies suggest that hydrogenated fats are more likely to raise blood cholesterol levels and should be used sparingly. Choose margarines, oils, and shortenings that list liquid vegetable oil as the first ingredient and that contain no more than 2 gm of saturated fatty acids per tablespoon (this information is found on the package or label).

Heart-healthy alternatives are polyunsaturated and monounsaturated fatty acids, which are mainly in liquid oils from these plants:

Polyunsaturated	**Monounsaturated**
Safflower seeds	Canola
Sesame seeds	Olives
Sunflower seeds	Peanuts
Corn and soybeans	Avocados
Nuts and seeds	

Both polyunsaturated and monounsaturated fatty acids may help lower your blood cholesterol level when the amount of **saturated** fatty acids in your diet is low. Keep in mind, however, these are still fats and should be used sparingly.

The American Heart Association has issued the following guidelines for lowering cholesterol and fat in your diet:

- Limit cholesterol to no more than 300 mg/day.
- Eat no more than 3 or 4 egg yolks a week, including those used in cooking (egg whites are healthy and a good source of protein).
- Eat no more than 6 oz of cooked lean meat, poultry, fish, or seafood a day.
- Reduce your total fat intake to no more than 30% of your total daily calories. Total fat should be less than 65 gm/day.
- Limit your intake of saturated fatty acids to less than 10% of total daily calories, or less than 20 gm/day.

You can reduce your blood cholesterol level by cutting down on high-fat foods and eating more of the following:

- Fruits, vegetables, and whole grains
- Fish, poultry without skin, and lean meats (trim all fat before cooking)
- Low fat or skim milk dairy products

DIETARY FAT

Fat should make up no more than 30% of the total calories in your diet. Total dietary fat should be split, roughly equally, among the three main types of fat: polyunsaturated, monounsaturated, and saturated.

DAILY CALORIE INTAKE	MAXIMUM FAT INTAKE PER DAY	
	In Calories	In Grams
1000	300	33
1200	360	40
1400	420	47
1600	480	53
1800	540	60
2000	600	67

Dietary fat is measured in units called grams. One gram of fat supplies 9 calories. If you eat a food that contains 5 gm of fat, you are eating 45 calories of fat in that serving (5 gm of fat × 9 calories/gm = 45 calories of fat).

CHOLESTEROL

Starting at age 20, have your cholesterol level checked and monitor this measurement throughout your life. Your doctor uses a blood test to measure your **total** blood cholesterol, HDL ("good"), and LDL ("bad") cholesterol levels. Another fat that is associated with increased risk for heart attack is triglycerides, and this level can be measured with the same test. The goal is to increase HDL and reduce LDL and triglyceride levels. The following classifications are used to identify high-risk persons and serve as guidelines for healthy cholesterol levels:

TOTAL BLOOD (SERUM) CHOLESTEROL

Desirable	Less than 200 mg/dl
Borderline high	200-239 mg/dl
High	240 mg/dl or higher

HDL (FOR WOMEN)

Desirable	50-60 mg/dl
Too low	35 mg/dl

LDL CHOLESTEROL

Desirable	Less than 130 mg/dl
Borderline high	130-159 mg/dl
High	160 mg/dl or higher

TRIGLYCERIDE LEVELS

Normal	Less than 200 mg/dl
Borderline high	200-399 mg/dl
High	400-999 mg/dl
Very high	1000 mg/dl or higher

KEEPING TABS ON HOMOCYSTEINE

Recent scientific studies suggest that homocysteine, an amino acid in the blood, could be associated with heart disease. Control of homocysteine levels can be achieved by maintaining an optimal daily intake of B vitamins and folic acid. The optimal daily intake of 3 to 3.5 mg of vitamin B_6, 350 to 400 μg of folic acid, and 5 to 15 μg of vitamin B_{12} will help to reduce the level of homocysteine. Most multivitamins contain these amounts.

RESOURCES

Notes

Notes

NOTES

Calendar

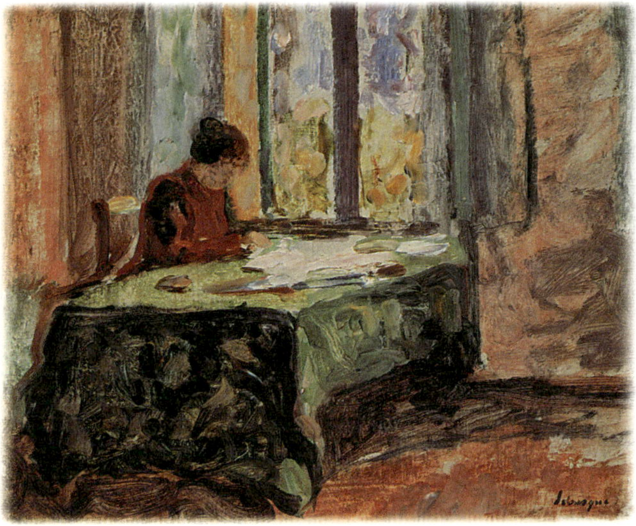

Femme Cousant

Lebasque, Henri (1865-1937)
French
Christie's
London

Calendar

Menstrual Record

YEAR: ____________

MONTH	1	2	3	4	5	6	7	8	9	10	11	12	13	14	15	16	17	18	19	20	21	22	23	24	25	26	27	28	29	30	31
JANUARY																															
FEBRUARY																															
MARCH																															
APRIL																															
MAY																															
JUNE																															
JULY																															
AUGUST																															
SEPTEMBER																															
OCTOBER																															
NOVEMBER																															
DECEMBER																															

TYPE OF FLOW

- ☒ NORMAL
- ☐ EXCEPTIONALLY LIGHT
- ■ EXCEPTIONALLY HEAVY
- ⊙ SPOTTING

Don't forget to have this chart with you when you call or visit your doctor.

Menstrual Record

YEAR: ______________

MONTH	1	2	3	4	5	6	7	8	9	10	11	12	13	14	15	16	17	18	19	20	21	22	23	24	25	26	27	28	29	30	31
JANUARY																															
FEBRUARY																															
MARCH																															
APRIL																															
MAY																															
JUNE																															
JULY																															
AUGUST																															
SEPTEMBER																															
OCTOBER																															
NOVEMBER																															
DECEMBER																															

TYPE OF FLOW

- ☒ **NORMAL**
- **EXCEPTIONALLY LIGHT**
- **EXCEPTIONALLY HEAVY**
- **SPOTTING**

Don't forget to have this chart with you when you call or visit your doctor.

Notes

MONTHLY REMINDERS

MONTH: YEAR:

MONDAY	TUESDAY	WEDNESDAY

Reminders:

- BREAST SELF-EXAMINATION
- DOCTOR'S VISITS
- OVULATION

THURSDAY	FRIDAY	SATURDAY	SUNDAY

Monthly Reminders

MONTH: YEAR:

MONDAY	TUESDAY	WEDNESDAY

Reminders:

- BREAST SELF-EXAMINATION
- DOCTOR'S VISITS
- OVULATION

THURSDAY	FRIDAY	SATURDAY	SUNDAY

Monthly Reminders

MONTH: YEAR:

MONDAY	TUESDAY	WEDNESDAY

Reminders:

- BREAST SELF-EXAMINATION
- DOCTOR'S VISITS
- OVULATION

THURSDAY	FRIDAY	SATURDAY	SUNDAY

Monthly Reminders

MONTH: YEAR:

MONDAY	TUESDAY	WEDNESDAY

Reminders:

- BREAST SELF-EXAMINATION
- DOCTOR'S VISITS
- OVULATION

THURSDAY	FRIDAY	SATURDAY	SUNDAY

Monthly Reminders

MONTH: YEAR:

MONDAY	TUESDAY	WEDNESDAY

Reminders:

- BREAST SELF-EXAMINATION
- DOCTOR'S VISITS
- OVULATION

THURSDAY	FRIDAY	SATURDAY	SUNDAY

Monthly Reminders

MONTH: YEAR:

Reminders:

- BREAST SELF-EXAMINATION
- DOCTOR'S VISITS
- OVULATION

MONDAY	TUESDAY	WEDNESDAY

THURSDAY	FRIDAY	SATURDAY	SUNDAY

MONTHLY REMINDERS

MONTH: YEAR:

MONDAY	TUESDAY	WEDNESDAY

Reminders:

- BREAST SELF-EXAMINATION
- DOCTOR'S VISITS
- OVULATION

THURSDAY	FRIDAY	SATURDAY	SUNDAY

MONTHLY REMINDERS

MONTH: YEAR:

Reminders:

- BREAST SELF-EXAMINATION
- DOCTOR'S VISITS
- OVULATION

MONDAY	TUESDAY	WEDNESDAY

THURSDAY	FRIDAY	SATURDAY	SUNDAY

Monthly Reminders

MONTH: YEAR:

Reminders:

- BREAST SELF-EXAMINATION
- DOCTOR'S VISITS
- OVULATION

MONDAY	TUESDAY	WEDNESDAY

THURSDAY	FRIDAY	SATURDAY	SUNDAY

Monthly Reminders

MONTH: YEAR:

MONDAY	TUESDAY	WEDNESDAY

Reminders:

- BREAST SELF-EXAMINATION
- DOCTOR'S VISITS
- OVULATION

THURSDAY	FRIDAY	SATURDAY	SUNDAY

Monthly Reminders

MONTH: YEAR:

Reminders:

- BREAST SELF-EXAMINATION
- DOCTOR'S VISITS
- OVULATION

MONDAY	TUESDAY	WEDNESDAY

THURSDAY	FRIDAY	SATURDAY	SUNDAY

Monthly Reminders

MONTH: YEAR:

MONDAY	TUESDAY	WEDNESDAY

Reminders:

- BREAST SELF-EXAMINATION
- DOCTOR'S VISITS
- OVULATION

THURSDAY	FRIDAY	SATURDAY	SUNDAY

Monthly Reminders

MONTH: YEAR:

MONDAY	TUESDAY	WEDNESDAY

Reminders:

- BREAST SELF-EXAMINATION
- DOCTOR'S VISITS
- OVULATION

THURSDAY	FRIDAY	SATURDAY	SUNDAY

Monthly Reminders

MONTH: YEAR:

Reminders:

- BREAST SELF-EXAMINATION
- DOCTOR'S VISITS
- OVULATION

MONDAY	TUESDAY	WEDNESDAY

THURSDAY	FRIDAY	SATURDAY	SUNDAY

MONTHLY REMINDERS

MONTH: YEAR:

MONDAY	TUESDAY	WEDNESDAY

Reminders:

- BREAST SELF-EXAMINATION
- DOCTOR'S VISITS
- OVULATION

THURSDAY	FRIDAY	SATURDAY	SUNDAY

Monthly Reminders

MONTH: YEAR:

MONDAY	TUESDAY	WEDNESDAY

Reminders:

- BREAST SELF-EXAMINATION
- DOCTOR'S VISITS
- OVULATION

THURSDAY	FRIDAY	SATURDAY	SUNDAY

Monthly Reminders

MONTH: YEAR:

MONDAY	TUESDAY	WEDNESDAY

Reminders:

- BREAST SELF-EXAMINATION
- DOCTOR'S VISITS
- OVULATION

THURSDAY	FRIDAY	SATURDAY	SUNDAY

Monthly Reminders

MONTH: YEAR:

MONDAY	TUESDAY	WEDNESDAY

Reminders:

- BREAST SELF-EXAMINATION
- DOCTOR'S VISITS
- OVULATION

THURSDAY	FRIDAY	SATURDAY	SUNDAY

NOTES

Kids' Notes

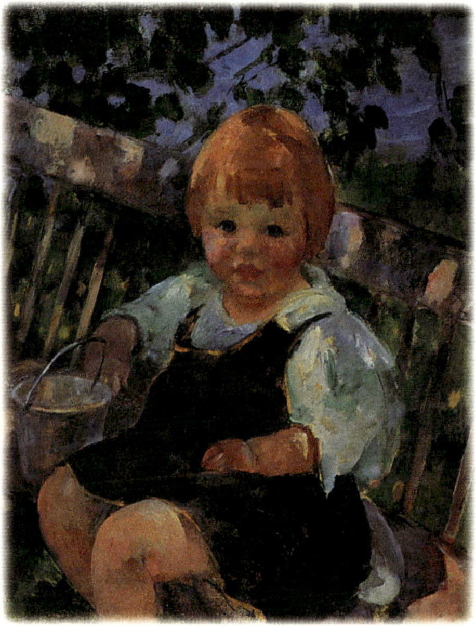

Red-Haired Child

Walter, Martha (1875-1976)
American
David David Gallery
Philadelphia, Pennsylvania

Kids' Notes

Kids' Notes

NAME:

PEDIATRICIAN:

PHONE:

DENTIST:

PHONE:

EYE DOCTOR:

PHONE:

PHARMACY:

PHONE:

DAYCARE:

PHONE:

SCHOOL:

PHONE:

BABYSITTER:

PHONE:

BABYSITTER:

PHONE:

FRIEND:

PHONE:

FRIEND:

PHONE:

FRIEND:

PHONE:

COACHES:

PHONE:

COACHES:

PHONE:

KIDS' NOTES

NAME:

PEDIATRICIAN:

PHONE:

DENTIST:

PHONE:

EYE DOCTOR:

PHONE:

PHARMACY:

PHONE:

DAYCARE:

PHONE:

SCHOOL:

PHONE:

BABYSITTER:

PHONE:

BABYSITTER:

PHONE:

FRIEND:

PHONE:

FRIEND:

PHONE:

FRIEND:

PHONE:

COACHES:

PHONE:

COACHES:

PHONE:

KIDS' NOTES

NAME:

PEDIATRICIAN:

PHONE:

DENTIST:

PHONE:

EYE DOCTOR:

PHONE:

PHARMACY:

PHONE:

DAYCARE:

PHONE:

SCHOOL:

PHONE:

BABYSITTER:

PHONE:

BABYSITTER:

PHONE:

FRIEND:

PHONE:

FRIEND:

PHONE:

FRIEND:

PHONE:

COACHES:

PHONE:

COACHES:

PHONE:

Kids' Notes

NAME:

PEDIATRICIAN:

PHONE:

DENTIST:

PHONE:

EYE DOCTOR:

PHONE:

PHARMACY:

PHONE:

DAYCARE:

PHONE:

SCHOOL:

PHONE:

BABYSITTER:

PHONE:

BABYSITTER:

PHONE:

FRIEND:

PHONE:

FRIEND:

PHONE:

FRIEND:

PHONE:

COACHES:

PHONE:

COACHES:

PHONE:

KIDS' NOTES

NAME:

PEDIATRICIAN:

PHONE:

DENTIST:

PHONE:

EYE DOCTOR:

PHONE:

PHARMACY:

PHONE:

DAYCARE:

PHONE:

SCHOOL:

PHONE:

BABYSITTER:

PHONE:

BABYSITTER:

PHONE:

FRIEND:

PHONE:

FRIEND:

PHONE:

FRIEND:

PHONE:

COACHES:

PHONE:

COACHES:

PHONE:

Kids' Notes

NAME:

PEDIATRICIAN:

PHONE:

DENTIST:

PHONE:

EYE DOCTOR:

PHONE:

PHARMACY:

PHONE:

DAYCARE:

PHONE:

SCHOOL:

PHONE:

BABYSITTER:

PHONE:

BABYSITTER:

PHONE:

FRIEND:

PHONE:

FRIEND:

PHONE:

FRIEND:

PHONE:

COACHES:

PHONE:

COACHES:

PHONE:

NOTES

NOTES

Telephone Numbers

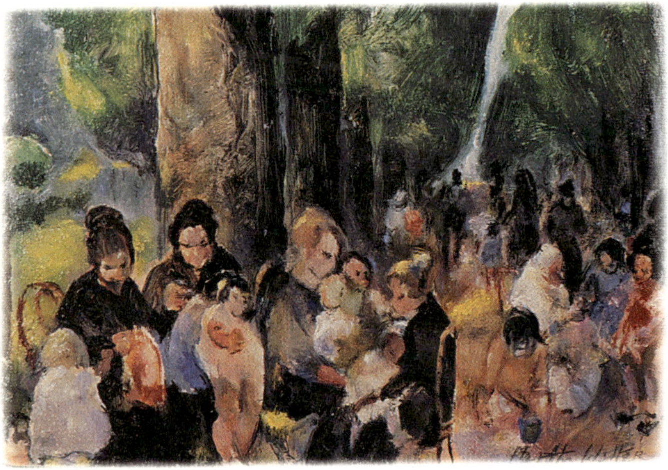

Luxembourg Gardens

Walter, Martha (1875-1976)
American
David David Gallery
Philadelphia, Pennsylvania

Phone • Fax • E-Mail Numbers

NAME	PHONE • FAX • E-MAIL

Phone • Fax • E-mail Numbers

NAME	PHONE • FAX • E-MAIL

Phone • Fax • E-mail Numbers

NAME	PHONE • FAX • E-MAIL

Phone • Fax • E-mail Numbers

NAME	PHONE • FAX • E-MAIL

Phone • Fax • E-mail Numbers

NAME	PHONE • FAX • E-MAIL

Phone • Fax • E-mail Numbers

NAME	PHONE • FAX • E-MAIL